Ten Ways to Kill a Pastor

Ten Ways to KILL A PASTOR

Reverend Christopher I. Thoma

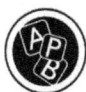

Angels' Portion Books

Text © 2016 by Christopher I. Thoma

FIRST EDITION, 2016

Angels' Portion Books
AngelsPortion.com

Images:
Cover, Five, Six, Seven, & Nine licensed by ShutterStock
Introduction, One through Four, Eight, Ten, & A Last Word by Jennifer A. Thoma
Nave Windows by Rebecca Molnar

For more information visit:
www.angelsportion.com

Cataloging-in-Publication Data
Thoma, Christopher I., 1972—
        Ten Ways to Kill a Pastor / Reverend Christopher
        I. Thoma – 1st Angels' Portion Books ed.
        ISBN-13: 978-1734186123
        1. Pastor/minister   2. Christian theology   3.
        Narrative 4. Fiction/non-fiction I. Title.
        APB 2019; Religion > Christian Life > Spiritual
        Warfare.

Printed in the United States of America

ENDORSEMENTS

❖

"Sharing experiences is important. The sharing of experience isn't to stop. And while seminary courses, fieldwork, and vicarage assignments all serve important roles in forming pastors for dealing with people, Chris Thoma brings together and shares the often-unteachable experiences in *Ten Ways to Kill a Pastor*. A Lutheran minister, Thoma faces off with ten troubling situations that often confront pastors and their families, and he does so through easy-to-read vignettes. Each is presented so vividly that the reader—whether pastor, spouse, or layperson—will ask silently, 'How is it that he knows me so well?' They are incredibly real and reflect life in the ministry from a very important perspective. Each chapter being a mirror of a pastor's soul, I highly recommend this as a resource to be studied and discussed by pastors and laypeople alike. The Lutheran Confessions speak of the 'mutual consolation of the brethren.' Thoma has provided a place where the need for that consolation can be identified and the effort begun."

REV. DR. DAVID P. SCAER
Chairman of the Systematics Department
Concordia Theological Seminary, Fort Wayne, Indiana
Author of *Discourses in Matthew* and
James: The Apostle of Faith

"This book provides a real and gritty depiction of the pastoral ministry. Pastor Thoma does a great service to the church by exposing the abuses that many pastors often endure while presenting the ever-present comfort of Christ Jesus. There is tremendous comfort—even in the midst of tremendous pain—knowing that God is not at war with His people."

REV. A. TREVOR SUTTON
Pastor of Saint Luke Lutheran Church
Haslett, Michigan
Author of *Being Lutheran*

"It is difficult for many church members to fully understand the demands of pastoral ministry. Chris Thoma helps by presenting ten high-stress scenarios caused by congregations that have the potential for destroying pastors."

KENT CROCKETT
President, Making Life Count Ministries, Inc.
Author of *Pastor Abusers: When Sheep Attack their Shepherd*
www.makinglifecount.net

"A defibrillator that delivers a therapeutic jolt of truth straight to the Christian heart!"

REV. TYREL BRAMWELL
Pastor of St. Mark Lutheran Church, Ferndale, California
Author of *The Gift and the Defender*

FOR
those who have suffered

❖

WHEN GOD WANTS to strengthen a man's faith He first weakens it by feigning to break faith within him. He thrusts him into many tribulations and makes him so weary that he is driven to despair, and yet He gives him strength to be still and persevere. Such quietness is perseverance, and perseverance produces experience, so that when God returns to him and lets His sun rise and shine again, and when the storm is over the man opens his eyes in amazement and says: "The Lord shall be praised, that I have been delivered...."

Within a day or two, within a week or a year, or even within the next hour, sin brings another cross to us: the loss of honor or possessions, bodily injury or some mishap which brings such trouble. Then it all begins again and the storm breaks out once more. But now we glory in our afflictions because we remember that on the former occasion God was gracious to us, and we know that it is His good will to chastise us, that we may have reason to run to Him and cry, "He who has helped me before, please help me now." And that self-same longing in your heart (which makes you cry, Oh that I were free! Oh that God would come! Oh that I might receive help!) is hope, which does not put to shame, for God must help such a person.

In this way God hides life in death, heaven under hell, wisdom under folly, and grace in our sin.

Martin Luther, *Sermons from the year 1527*

CONTENTS

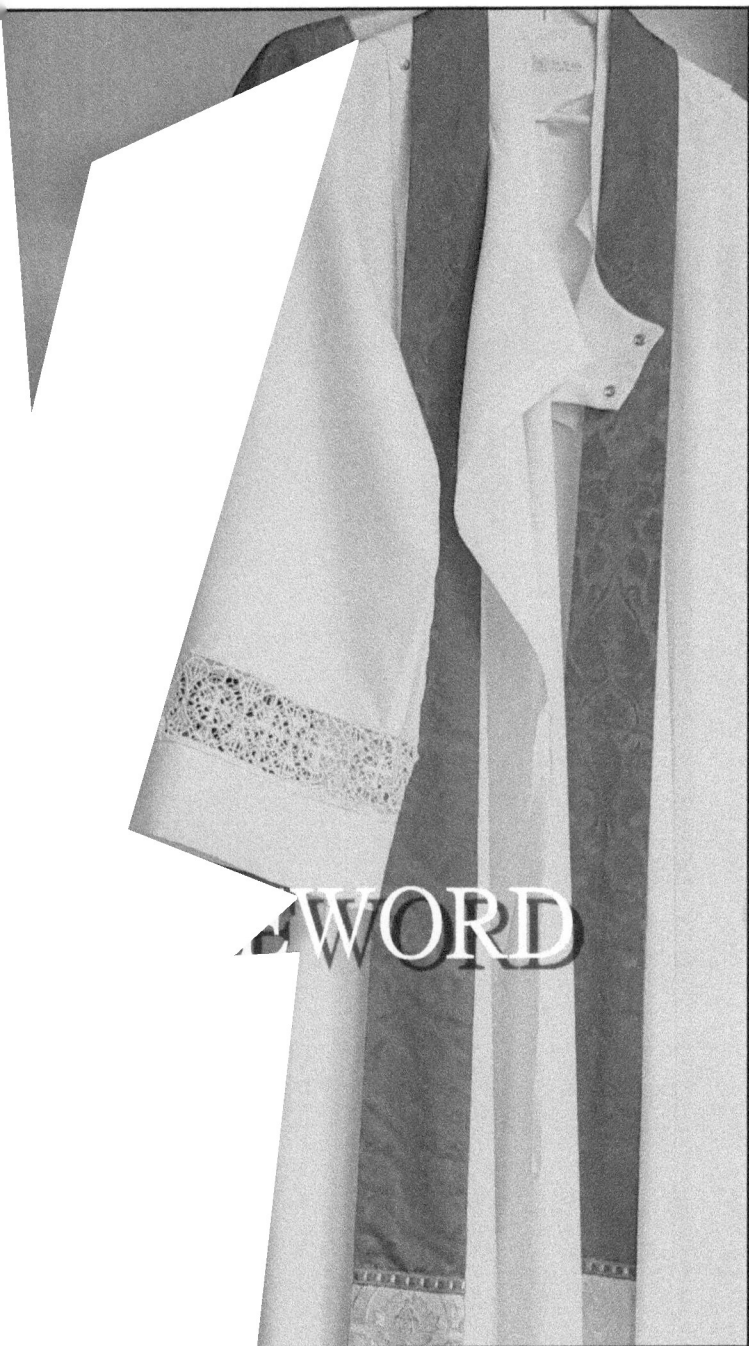

EWORD

FOREWORD

❖

MOST MEN WHO enter the seminary have no idea concerning the challenges that await. Generally, they come with a healthy fear of learning the languages of Hebrew and Greek. They realize the academic acumen will be "kicked up a notch" or two. They even lay awake at night, wondering if they will survive their first sermon delivery without throwing up or falling out of the pulpit. But the majority has no clue as to the challenges and dangers of the pastoral office.

In these days and times, there is an inherent understanding that things will get rough out there. The signs of the times are clear enough to signal a new day for ministry that will most certainly test the mettle of the most stalwart of clergy. Gender issues, or lack thereof; government mandates and demands concerning marriage and family; court-ordered compliances; accusations of hate speech from the pulpit—these all loom on the not-so-distant horizon. These things are mostly known and understood as the "new normal" for the Church of God and her called servants. These things within this reality are what we tend to focus upon. It is what is known and expected as men bravely enter into the Office of the Public Ministry.

But there are other, even greater, dangers and challenges. These do not come from the world outside; they lurk within the walls. Within the very walls of the church itself, there are many and various dangers to the pastor and his family. The people of God, the family of the church, can be a perilous group. So many personalities, so many issues past and present, scar tissue from the previous troubles, family dynamics that wage war using the church as a battlefield…and it is into this eclectic mix that a pastor is called. And, as a pastor, the expectation is that he will solve and soothe, rally, adjudicate, motivate and navigate the church through these tumultuous waters.

As the placement director at Concordia Theological Seminary in Fort Wayne, Indiana I know two things for certain. The first is that *NO PASTOR* can deal with these strange and peculiar dynamics that exist within every church, and there are no self-help books or magic wands available at the seminary bookstore that will provide the secret or the cure. The second thing I know is that *NO CHURCH* calls a pastor with the desire or goal to destroy him and his family. It is true that some churches have a rather checkered track record, but this is not the goal or desire. As Pastor Thoma points out, fear and ignorance immobilize and cripple the ministry. Satan worms his way into the church and plants these seeds and only Christ through His holy Word and precious Sacraments can overcome.

Pastor Thoma has provided ten stories written with his unique style and grace that not only help illustrate the problems but also pull each of us into the fray. And, as we see ourselves as abused or abusers, we also see the need for the One who endured all things that we might be "Church" in the truest sense of the word.

The reading will be easy, the swallowing will be hard—continue on to *A Last Word*.

Rev. Dr. Jeffrey H. Pulse
Professor of Exegetical Theology & Director of Certification and Placement
Concordia Theological Seminary

INTRODUCTION

INTRODUCTION

❖

I DON'T REMEMBER ever wanting or expecting to write a book like this, and yet the viscera of the manuscript before you took only five days to spill.

These stories were far too easy to tell.

Additionally, I don't recall any particular class at the seminary in which the professor, an experienced parish pastor now garnished with doctoral degrees, stood before me and my classmates to warn us that even though we'd set our hearts upon on a very noble task (1 Timothy 3:1), the endeavor might lead to indescribable stress and unspeakable abuse at the hands of those we were preparing to serve. It might even lead to our crucifixions, so to speak (John 16:2).

I don't remember that lecture.

I don't remember studying the subject in a textbook. I don't remember it as a topic of conversation around the community lunch table. I don't remember it being broached in vicarage or placement interviews. I don't remember any willful efforts to see that I would be ready—that I would know what to do when the alligators surfaced and the sharks started circling; that I would know where and when to go for help within the church's broader landscape of resources.

I just don't remember.

Still, Jesus didn't hold back on the detail that those standing in His stead and by His command would be found facing off with otherworldly forces (Luke 22:31; Ephesians 6:12), and not necessarily on approach from the church's borderlands, but quite often from within (Acts 20:28-31; 2 Timothy 4:3).

He warned us.

The book in your hands at this moment isn't designed to systematically list and then define the many and various things that people do metaphorically to kill their pastors. There are other volumes worthy of your attention that accomplish

24

this, most notably Kent Crockett's book entitled *Pastor Abusers: When Sheep Attack Their Shepherd.* The book before you now is different.

First and foremost, this volume is a collection of fictional short stories born from excruciating experience, each one dealing with a different pastor in a different congregation in a different place. By way of these stories, the effort is made to raise awareness among God's people by carrying the reader into and among challenges facing pastors and their families. It is framed in a way that allows you to observe the unobservable. It works to set you into stride beside the one called by Christ to preach His Gospel and administer His gifts, and it does so by consenting to you the darker involvements of the calling. It gives a voice—a narrative—to the things a pastor experiences but rarely shares.

This book also serves, in a sense, as a certain measure of consolation to pastors who are or have been subject to abuse. It tells the stories they already know so well and, by doing so, affirms a particular reality: others have been there. You are not alone.

Finally, it carries in its heart the desire to take seriously the cratered and bloody landscape that exists between the darkness of the Church Militant and the daylight of forever in the Church Triumphant. Some of the stories will be harder to read than others. Nevertheless, I encourage you to take them into yourself, and as you do, to remember that which is most important: The Gospel.

The Gospel shows you that even as the storm clouds begin to gather and the horizon becomes dark, God is good, and no matter what happens, the giving of His Son into death for the forgiveness of sins forever demonstrates His goodness and reminds even the most oppressed that He is not at war with His people (Romans 5:1-5). That war ended at Calvary with the words "It is finished" (John 19:30). He loves you, and He is, even now, working all things for your salvation according to His good and gracious will (Romans 8:28-39; John 6:38-40).

Pastors, be secured by this. You have the assurance from Christ Himself that He will never leave you nor forsake you. He is with you on the battlefield. He is near to you amid the cindering haze. He is there to strengthen and shield you by the power of His Gospel and to dress the wounds of human doubt, foolishness, and despair with the same.

The message of Jesus Christ and Him crucified is the affirming proclamation of this immeasurable love. Look to this and hold it close. It is the divine muscle for life through and after the struggles—no matter where they end. It is the marvelously pure oxygen that fills your lungs so that you might endure and declare:

> "The LORD is my light and my salvation;
>> whom shall I fear?
> The LORD is the stronghold of my life;
>> of whom shall I be afraid?
> When evildoers assail me
>> to eat up my flesh,
> my adversaries and foes,
>> it is they who stumble and fall.
> Though an army encamp against me,
>> my heart shall not fear;
> though war arise against me,
>> yet I will be confident."
>> (Psalm 27:1-3)

"...and they shall become one flesh."
Matthew 5:37

ONE

The Pastor's
Wife

❖

I T WAS LATE. The drive home was quiet.

After a while, the hum from the road became an uneasy song and so he reached for the radio. She fixed her gaze through the window into the nothingness of the farmlands palled by the evening, every now and then eyeing a weathered barn or a snow covered scarecrow.

"The Tackletons have a nice home," he said and fixed the radio on a classic rock station, being sure to keep the volume low. "They really seem to get into the Christmas spirit."

"Yeah, they do," she replied. "Beautiful." The station fizzed a little as they passed beneath a power line. It started to snow.

"Jim mentioned that he'd come over this week to fix the bathroom sink in the parsonage," he added, tapping unnecessarily at the tuner.

"That's nice," she said. "He seems nice."

"I told him Tuesday would be best," he said, filling in the empty air space. "That seemed best since Monday is busy with Emily and Sarah's dance class."

"That's fine," she mumbled.

"I figure he can come over after the council meeting, as long as it doesn't go too long."

"Whatever. That's fine." The snow was getting heavier. As he slowed, the road hum turned to a frapping of wet snow in the wheel wells of their struggling Ford.

"You okay?" he asked and reached for her hand. He knew it had been a difficult night. She shied from his approach momentarily but then relaxed and grasped in return.

"I'm fine," she said, finally glancing at him. "It was a long night. I just want to get home."

"Yeah," he chuckled uneasily. "My face actually hurts from trying to smile so much."

"Yeah…"

The next few miles were a slow junket of steady snow and Bob Segar. And then she spoke.

"I have a name, you know," she said abruptly. Before he could respond, she turned to him and repeated, "I have a name. It's Lynn. My name is Lynn."

He didn't say anything. He kept his eyes on the road and listened.

"No one ever calls me by my name," she sighed. "To everyone at that party, I wasn't Lynn. I was your wife. I was 'Pastor's wife.'"

He attempted to speak, but she kept on.

"And they don't even look at me when we're together,' she said, turning back to the window. "They talk to you. They ask you things. They barely even acknowledge I'm there."

"Give it some time, honey," he tried. The snow was getting worse. "We're new. They're still getting to know us. They're still getting to know you."

"We've been here since August," she argued. "It's been five months."

"It'll change," he said. "It'll get better. Maybe you could get involved, maybe volunteer to lead the…"

"No, I'm not volunteering! And no, it won't get better!" she snapped. "Just because I'm the pastor's wife doesn't mean I need to teach Sunday school,

33

lead a Bible study, or join the quilting group. I don't want to do those things. I don't have time to do things like that. I'm a mother. I work full-time at the bank. You're never around. I barely have time to take care of everything else in our lives. I'm not going to give away the little time that I have and need to be a faithful mother to our kids—to us.

"Yes, I know, but I think—"

"Don't," she interrupted. "Just don't."

The wipers were pounding the windshield.

"I know you think I sound selfish," she said shakily. "And I know you probably think I'm making something from nothing. But you need to know that I don't want to be the pastor's wife and that's it. I want to be Lynn, too. I want to be me."

She started to cry just as he turned the wheel and stopped the car in their driveway. The garage light struggled against the sizeable snowflakes casting thick shadows on the ground. He turned to take her hand again, but this time she refused and got out of the car. He moved quickly to intercept her on the porch. Taking her in his arms, he held her close.

"I love you," he said. "We're in this together. And I'll do whatever it takes to change this for you."

"I know," she said and tucked herself into the collar of his coat. "But it's hard to change what is."

The babysitter flipped on the porch light and peeked through the living room window. The pastor and the pastor's wife embraced.

Each could see the other's breath in the cold.

"Let what you say be simply 'Yes' or 'No';
anything more than this comes from evil."

Matthew 5:37

Two

Anonymous

❖

HE DIDN'T NOTICE it until he was already in the car. A busy day of services and Bible studies behind him, he was the last to leave and anxious to get home. The note was tucked into a yellow envelope and pinned to the windshield by the driver's side wiper blade. "From A Friend" was written on the outside.

He opened his door just enough to put one foot on the ground and then reached around to retrieve the missive.

"I'm glad it didn't rain," he whispered. "It looked like rain all morning."

He opened the letter.

Dear Pastor,

I've been wanting to write this letter for some time now. I guess I finally worked up the courage to do it.

I want to start by telling you that I think you are a great pastor and value our friendship. I really do, which is why I'm writing this letter. I hope you will take what I have to say to heart and that you will at least consider my words, not just because they come from someone who cares about you and your family, but because I'm not the only one who feels this way. I've had several conversations with others, and I can tell you that they feel the same way.

I think how you handled the situation with Jim Slater's son Caleb was wrong, and let me tell you why.

We are a small congregation. The budget is tight, and we can't afford to lose families. Refusing to commune Caleb because he and his fiancée are living together wasn't helpful. I spoke with Jim and Kathy after church last week, and they said they're thinking about leaving and going to the Methodist church in town. And they mentioned that Caleb's sister, Penny, and her husband are thinking about it, too. I'm really concerned about this, Pastor.

I know you met with Caleb and his fiancée in private (sorry, I don't know her name, but she seems like a nice enough girl).

Jim told me about the meeting. He said Caleb told him that all you pretty much did was use Bible verses to talk down to them. I don't know if you did or if you didn't. I wasn't there. And I guess Jim wasn't either, but still, I think you should have considered that they're getting married in a couple of months at her church. That's good for something, right? It seems like they have the right intentions, and I'd say that the whole problem will be solved on its own this fall. It just doesn't seem like it needs to be something that offends a pillar family in the congregation.

I'm not sure if you know it or not, but Jim had a hand in building this church. He spearheaded the building campaign and was the guy who negotiated the deal for the land. And Kathy has been the Sunday school superintendent here since long before you ever arrived. The Slaters are good people. We owe them a lot for all they've done over the years. I would hate to see them leave because of something that really does seem pretty small.

I hope you will reconsider what you've done and how you've handled the situation and maybe be encouraged by this note to think about apologizing to the Slaters and Caleb and his future wife. I don't know if it will make much of a difference now because they seem pretty intent upon leaving, but Jim's a friend of mine, just like you, and I don't like seeing him so down. He's hurting, Pastor. Their whole family is hurting. An apology from you might be all it takes to help to start the healing process.

I should add that if the Slaters leave, it will be a hard thing for me and my family to swallow and would most likely affect our relationship with this congregation, too. I don't want that. I really don't.

Please pray about this, Pastor, and as I said, I hope you'll take my words to heart and do the right thing to turn this situation around. You can count on me, as a friend, to pray for you, too.

Yours in Jesus,
A Friend

He slowly folded the letter at its predefined creases, giving each pleat a slow swipe, and then put it back into the envelope. Still holding it, he started his car and sat still for a moment.

Staring out the window toward a somewhat overcast sky, he gave a sigh. He set the letter in the passenger seat and lifted his foot from the brake just enough for the car to roll forward in a crawl. At the parking lot's exit, he stopped, and although the highway was barren in both directions, he looked back and forth as though he either didn't know which way he would go or was waiting for his opportunity to engage in the invisible traffic's flow.

And then he looked straight ahead.

"It looked like rain all morning," he whispered again while tapping the steering wheel and examining the ditch beyond the roadway.

Giving another sigh, he turned left out of the lot and went home.

THREE

"But Peter said, 'Man, I do not know what you are talking about.' And immediately while he was still speaking, the rooster crowed. And the Lord turned and looked at Peter..."

Luke 22:60, 61

The Clandestine Agenda

❖

"HEY, BILL, YOU got a minute?" Tom asked, putting his arm around his longtime friend's shoulder.

"Sure," he offered. "What's up?"

Leaving the wives to chat in the hallway, Tom shepherded Bill into a nearby Sunday school classroom where a small number of others were already sipping coffee and waiting.

"Uh-oh," Bill chuckled somewhat uneasily as Tom closed the door behind him. "I'm guessing it's something serious."

"Well, sort of," Tom said, scratching his chin and looking at the floor.

"What is it?"

"I'm just curious," Tom said in a softer tone. "What do you think of Pastor?"

"What do you mean?"

A brief moment of silence passed.

"We think," Tom started and then shifted his gaze to the others in the room, "he's doing a lot more wrong than he is right and he needs to go."

It was easy to see that Bill, a soft-spoken and well-respected member of the parish, and a close friend of the pastor, had a genuine look of surprise. It was, indeed, an unexpected topic of conversation they'd set before him.

Bill took a breath to speak but was immediately interrupted by one voice and then another and then another until all in the room were adding individual pieces to a litany of not only the pastor's proposed failings, but what they felt were his deliberate offenses—one of which was described as having risen to the level of measured deceit.

"He lied, Bill," Tom said. "I know you're friends with him, but he lied."

"He did?!"

"Yes, he did."

"About what?"

"Well," Tom said and briefly looked away, "I don't think it's appropriate to reveal those details just yet."

But Bill had never seen or experienced his friend and pastor exhibiting the behaviors described by the people surrounding him. Not once. And yet those same people standing before him and working so hard to convince him were folks that he'd known for years, some even for decades—fellow Christians with whom he'd worshipped, vacationed, played softball, gone camping, celebrated baptisms and birthdays and confirmations and graduations. Certainly, their concerns were valid. Certainly, their experiences indicated something happening behind the scenes, something he hadn't seen yet. Why would they lie? Why would they all lie?

Carol, Tom's wife, tapped on the classroom window and pointed to her watch. The door muffled her voice, but it was clear enough to understand that the couple was running late for an after-church event. Tom waved her away.

Barbara, Bill's wife, tapped on the window and gave Bill a look. Bill smiled, "I'll be there in a second."

"We don't want a mess here, Bill," Tom said, looking at his watch and betraying his desire to conclude the meeting. "We want what's best for this church, and what's best is to get rid of this guy. And we thought that if enough of us are willing to speak up and share our common concerns, others will listen and follow our lead."

"And then what happens?" Bill asked.

"Well, only the good Lord knows for sure," Tom said without hesitation. "I, for one, am willing to approach Pastor Johnson and tell him that he should consider resigning."

"Yeah, I don't know, Tom. Maybe we should…"

"It's best not to tiptoe around this stuff," Tom said crisply, shifting his stance toward the door. "Unless, of course, someone else wants to talk to him. It might not hurt if more than one of us went to him in private. It'll make it clear to him that the concerns are congregation-wide." Another in the room said she would be willing to stop by his office for a visit.

"I'll call him tonight," Bill said. "He's a friend. And Saint Paul said not to let the sun go down on this kind of stuff, or something like that. Besides, I don't like to sit on these kinds of things for too long, anyways."

Everyone in the room nodded in agreement. But not Bill. He looked at the floor. His heart was beating swiftly, but it was also breaking. He couldn't believe what was happening. He was wishing that he hadn't followed Tom into the room.

"Would you mind giving me a quick call after you talk with him, Bill?" Tom asked. "But don't call till after 7:00. Nancy and I are watching the grandkids tonight. Mike and Jeanie are celebrating their anniversary."

"Sure, I can call."

"Thanks. And then I'll call him tomorrow and maybe see if he wants to get coffee in town."

The group filed from the room, some thanking others for their faithfulness.

On the way home, Bill said a silent prayer. Barbara asked him about the impromptu meeting, but he was too bothered to explain it properly. Once home, while Barbara was making lunch, he did his best to retell the story. He was surprised by her relatively passive response.

"I'm glad you're reaching out to him first," she said. "He needs to hear this from someone who cares about him."

"I don't think that's going to matter too much, Barbara," he said, putting his hands on his face and then wiping them up and over the top of his receding hair. "It doesn't matter who tells you something like this. It ain't what one wants to hear."

"No," she said. "It isn't."

Bill took a bite of his sandwich. He didn't feel like eating.

"I'd better call him now," he said with a mouth full of ham and cheese. "Think he's still at the church?"

"Most likely," she said. "It usually takes a while for him to get out of there."

Bill went to the phone and dialed the number. He knew it by heart. It rang only once.

"Hello, this is Pastor Johnson," spoke the kindly voice on the other end of the line.

"Hi, Pastor, it's Bill."

"Hey, Bill!" the voice sing-songed with sincerity. "Long time no talk, my friend."

"Yeah, it's been a while, Pastor," he returned with an uncomfortable chuckle.

"What can I do for you?"

"Say," he said, rubbing his forehead, "do you have a minute to talk?"

FOUR

"And on the seventh day God finished his work that he had done, and he rested..."

Genesis 2:2

Exhaustion

❖

THIRTY-FOUR DAYS.

It had been thirty-four consecutive days since the last time he'd been home other than to shower, shave, and sleep. Sadly, his twenty-three-day record was now broken.

The season of Lent was in full flex and swiftly approaching Holy Week and Easter. The little church was suffering another of her increasingly common financial watersheds, and one of the teachers in the fledgling little church school had taken a new position and would be leaving at the end of the semester.

Numerous additional meetings across multiple boards and committees were both required and scheduled by their chairpersons, each consuming the only free evenings of his already thinned week. He was exhausted. He was looking forward to today, a Saturday with no demands, a full day at home with his wife and children.

Being an unusually warm day for early April, he poured himself a cup of late-morning coffee. He went outside to sit beside his wife, who was already situated on the bottom step of the deck, scrolling through newsfeeds on her phone. She had successfully convinced the children to trade their morning cartoons for the opportunity to play outside. They were orchestrating a rather animated game of freeze tag.

"How's the coffee?" she asked him as he took a sip.

"Good," he said. "It's the flavored stuff."

"But you don't like the flavored stuff."

"It's all we had in there," he said, smiling. "I took it out of that gift basket of snacks the Tackelton's gave us at Christmas. I figured it was about time to open it." He took another sip. "It's pumpkin spice."

"And the verdict?"

"It's gross," he said, smiling again, "but it does the trick." Putting his arm around her, "There's plenty left," he said. "Want me to pour you a cup?"

"Funny," she said, giving him a gentle jab to the ribs. She took advantage of his embrace and rested her head on his chest. "What do you want to do today?"

"Whatever you want. I'm just glad to be home."

"I thought we could take the kids to the indoor waterpark in Davis for a few hours. It's only a half hour away, and I think they'd love it."

"Sounds good," he said and took another sip. "What time do you want to leave?"

"How about after lunch?"

The phone in the kitchen began to ring. Neither moved to answer. A few minutes passed. The phone rang again. Still, they remained fixed. They could hear the muted tone of the phone's voicemail beep, followed by a man's voice leaving what seemed to be a rather lengthy message.

"I wonder who that was," he said and sipped again. "I'd better go check." He began to lift from his seat on the step when she put both arms around his waist and pulled him back down.

"Just leave it," she said. "You can check it when we get home from the waterpark. You're mine right now."

Just then, the phone in her hand started to vibrate. They both looked at the screen.

"It's Gabe," he said. "He must be trying you now since we didn't answer the house phone. I'll bet he already left a message on my phone."

"Do you want me to answer?"

"Yeah," he relented and set his coffee mug beside him. "Go ahead and see what he wants."

"Hello... Hi, Gabe... Yep, we're just sitting on the deck steps watching the kids... It sure is... Yes, it's a perfect day to be at home... Yeah, he's here. Hold on a sec, and I'll get him..." She handed the phone to her husband and then moved her ear next to his to listen.

"Hey, Gabe."

"Hi, Pastor. Hey, I'm sorry to bother you on your day off, but John asked me to get the agenda together for the meeting on Monday night. I just checked my email and saw I got about twenty candidate résumés from the district. I already forwarded them to you. Could you take some time today to go through them and make some notes so that I can make copies and get them to the rest of the committee members at church tomorrow?"

"Does it have to be today? Could I get them to you tomorrow after church, and then you could just email them out? That should give folks enough time to look them over."

"A couple of folks on the committee don't use email, and John's one of them. Also, he just called a little while ago, saying he's taking off for a quick trip up north to open up his cabin. He'll be at the Monday meeting, but he won't be at church tomorrow, so as soon as you have it ready, I thought I'd just take it over to him before he goes. He said he'd flip through 'em while he's up there."

"I'll do what I can, Gabe. That's quite a few candidates, and Jamie and I are just getting ready to leave with the kids soon."

"Well, like you said, do what you can. We've got some time. But I know if you get them to me by 3:00, we'll be in good shape."

"I'll do what I can. Thanks for calling."

"Thanks, Pastor. I'll watch for your email. Talk to you soon."

He handed the phone back to her. She was fuming and near the edge of tears.

"If I get started now," he said, "I might be able to get this together for him before we leave."

"C'mon inside, guys," she called to the kids. "We're going to eat lunch and head to the waterpark."

There was a flurry of excitement as the kids forced their way through the narrow space between Mom and Dad and bounded up and into the house. Before closing the door behind him, the youngest turned and asked, "Is daddy coming with us?"

"I don't know, honey," she said. "Maybe next time."

"For the Scripture says, 'You shall not muzzle an ox when it treads out the grain,' and, 'The laborer deserves his wages.'"

1 Timothy 5:18

FIVE

Muzzling the Ox

❖

OING HIS BEST to be quiet, he closed the front door carefully and then locked it. He didn't reach for the light switch but sat on the bench near the door to remove his shoes. He struggled yet remained unwilling to turn on the light. A few nights prior he'd learned the hard way that if the baby's bedroom door was accidentally left open, the hallway mirror reflected the entryway light into the room and onto the crib. Anna had asked him to take the mirror and hang it in the living room, but finding the time to do something so simple seemed challenging.

He'd get to it tomorrow. Always tomorrow.

With his black case in hand, he made his way into the only room with light. Anna was at the kitchen table; papers fanned to each of its four corners.

"There's leftover spaghetti in the fridge," she said, shuffled a few pages, and then jotted in the checkbook ledger. "It's in the dish with the red lid." She scratched another note. "How was the meeting?"

"Same as usual," he said and opened the refrigerator door. Reaching for the dish with the red lid, he continued, "We talked about everything and nothing." He passed the microwave and went straight to the silverware drawer. "Some folks just like to talk, I guess," he said, leaning against the counter.

"You don't want to heat that up?"

"Nah, it's fine. Thanks for saving it for me."

He said a quiet prayer and then took a bite.

"What's it looking like this month?" he asked with a mouthful of cold pasta.

"You really need to sit down and look at these numbers with me," she insisted. "I'm serious. I can't do this by myself."

"Where are we short?" he asked.

"We're short everywhere," she said with evident distress. "We have just enough for the mortgage, but not enough for the water bill."

"How long can we hold that one?"

"Maybe about ten days. But we're taking a chance if we do that again this month. Last time the shut-off notice came with a warning that if we missed the due date again, a thousand-dollar deposit would be required to continue service."

"Well then, we need to figure out how to pay that one. Are there any other bills we can hold back? How about the loans?" He took another bite. "Did we make the student loan payment this month? Or the car?"

She paged through the online banking statements on the table before her.

"Those were automatically withdrawn on the first of the month," she confirmed. "Those have been paid."

"What about cable? That's both the TV and the internet, right? Isn't that about $150 or so?"

"We don't have TV or internet anymore, honey," she said, handing him a copy of the cancellation letter she'd sent last month. "I canceled that already."

"You did?! I didn't know that."

"When was the last time you saw any of us watching TV?"

"I don't know," he said and pulled out a chair to her left to sit beside her. "I thought I saw the kids watching TV one night last week."

"They've been watching DVDs that we got from the library, Kurt. And besides, you were gone every night last week. You didn't see them doing anything except sleeping."

Doing his best to swerve and avoid a collision with what could have easily become another disheartening discussion, "Well, we could maybe cut back on the grocery bill this week by getting some things from the food pantry at the church."

"Yeah, we could do that," she said. "I just put a box full of soup cans and cereal boxes in there last week, stuff that the manager over at the Kroger gave me at half price. It expires pretty soon, but I figure it's got about a month left."

"How much would that..." he started to say before she interrupted him.

"But soup and cereal will only go so far in a family of five," she said, laying her head flat on her right arm on the table.

"We can make it work. God will provide. He always does."

Her head still resting on her arm, she shifted to her left arm and looked away to the family portraits hanging in the hallway. It was too hard to see the faces because of the darkness.

"Have you ever thought about asking the church council for a raise?" she asked still looking away.

"Honey, I…"

Sitting up and snapping back toward him, "It's been six years, Kurt. You're still getting paid what they gave you when you started."

"I know, but…"

"And why?" she asked angrily. "I'll tell you why. Because they're more interested in building a new church sign by the road, installing thousands of dollars of new sound equipment, and buying new appliances for the kitchen than seeing that you get paid a living wage—that you get what you'd be worth to any other church."

He sat back in his chair. He was no longer interested in the spaghetti.

"Honey, now is not the time to ask the council for more money," he said. "We both know that the church was in a bad way when we got here, and I'm working as hard as I can to get her to a place where all the bills get paid on time. It's taken a lot of work to—"

"—What about us, Kurt?" she asked. "The church isn't struggling! People drive around in brand-new cars and take vacations whenever and wherever they want. The church isn't struggling, Kurt! The people aren't giving! And they're balancing the shortfall on our backs. They're taking advantage of the fact that we won't complain, that

67

we'll simply trust the Lord and take whatever they give us."

"That's what I'm trying to change, Anna," he said. "I'm trying to lead them out of that old life. I'm trying to teach them the joy of trusting the Lord."

"Well, something needs to change soon because we can't do this anymore."

"What do you mean?"

"I mean I've already got two cleaning jobs that take up most of the day. I mean that I can't get another job. I mean that someone needs to be around to help the kids with homework, get them to bed, and help handle all this *ungodliness* spread across the table."

She pushed the papers away in a flurry and put her head in her hands. Some of the pages fell to the floor.

"You're always saying that God never forsakes His people," she continued, but now much quieter, "and that in the middle of struggles, we should use the reason and senses He's given to seek faithfulness to Him. I trust Him. I do. But maybe our reason and senses are telling us we need to leave this church. Maybe we need to go where you can be a pastor, not an indentured servant."

She took his hand and pleaded, "Please, Kurt. Just talk to the leadership. Talk to someone."

Her stare was piercing. More than any other time, he felt he wanted to resign, but not just from his pastorate.

He was failing her.

He was failing their children.

Was he failing the Lord?

"I will," he said and got up. Standing at the kitchen sink, he hunched over a little and added, "I'll call Bob in the morning and see if we can get the Board of Elders together for a quick meeting." He put his spaghetti dish in the sink. "They're good men," he said. "They'll understand."

"Thank you."

The room went silent.

"I'm sorry, Anna," he said quietly and started to cry, but she'd already left the room. He reached into the cabinet above the sink for a pill bottle—Paxil— but then pulled back before touching it. It was empty.

"Oh, right," he said, wiping away a forming tear. "Our copay is fifty dollars now."

Six

"Therefore encourage one another and build one another up..."

1 Thessalonians 5:11

The Pastor is to Blame

❖

THE DISTRICT BISHOP'S greeting was followed by a lengthy monologue that seemed to drone for quite some time before the young pastor was finally presented with the opportunity to respond. He could see his ordination photo on the shelf just beyond his computer screen. The Bishop had attended.

"Bishop," he spoke into the phone, "I certainly don't mean to question your judgment, but don't you think I should know who stopped in to see you?"

"Now, John," he said in his trademark grandfatherly voice, "I gave my word that I would maintain confidentiality."

"But it doesn't make much sense for me to be accused of something—that someone actually made an appointment with you to talk about me—and not to be able to try to talk it out with them—to reconcile."

"John, I was in the parish for twenty-two years before being elected to this position," he said. "I'm no spring chicken to these types of situations. These take time. It'll get worked out one way or the other."

"May I ask, then," the young pastor continued, "what the concern was they shared?"

"Hold on a second," the Bishop said. "Let me grab my notes from the meeting."

There was a moment of silence and then a distant rustling of paper. While the Bishop was retrieving his notes, John reached for pen and paper to jot his own.

"Ah, here we go," the Bishop grunted as though he were sitting back down in his chair. "The concerns were three-fold. First, you don't seem to be serving with the same level of effort as your predecessor. Second, you're making too many changes too quickly. And third, you're not very approachable."

"That's quite a few concerns," he said. "Did the person give you any examples?"

"Oh yes," he said. "I have a couple of pages of notes, here, and some of it is rather troublesome, which is why I called you."

"Am I allowed to know any of the specifics?"

"Well, for one," the Bishop began, "the person said that you're not exhibiting the same enthusiasm about the new building project that's currently underway. Your predecessor was very supportive, but you seem to be trying to undermine the whole process."

"Did the person explain why he or she was feeling that way?"

"It seems you are rather confrontational when you ask questions of various committees and that you're probing into areas where the building committee has already done a lot of work."

"Bishop," he responded, "this project was started by a handful of members. It was by no means a congregation-wide decision or effort. But all of us— the whole congregation—just took on a million-dollar building expense. Yet, we're dragging along twenty years of declining attendance and income. The effort has already started, but since the Lord has seen fit to allow it, I am working to support its success with all I have. Still, the congregation needs to understand the challenges and what they mean for the future."

"Yes, they do," he affirmed. "But you also need to trust the people God has put into place to move this thing forward."

"I do trust them," he said. "And I support them 100%. But I'm also the new guy. It's really easy to start a program and then leave. It's nearly impossible to come into one and try to lead when you don't know the details."

"Maybe just let them do their work. You worry about other things—which brings me to the second concern."

"Go ahead."

"I've seen this one before. A new pastor comes in, whether a rookie or a veteran, and he begins making changes. The rookie tries to make the changes that reflect the ideals he envisioned while at the seminary. The veteran tries to make the church into something similar to the congregation he just left."

"But I haven't made any changes," he said. "Not a single one."

"This person said you completely rearranged the worship bulletin and now it's harder for people to follow."

"I didn't change anything in the bulletin," he said. "It's the same one they've been using since, well, forever. The only difference is that I added a brief communion statement below the image on the front cover. The elders told me they'd bugged my predecessor to do it, but he never did. I thought it was a valid concern so I got right on it."

"Do you think you would have added it if you didn't think it was valid?"

"What do you mean?"

"Never mind," the Bishop said and shifted gears. "Speaking of the communion statement, this person did mention it and said that it's written in a way that sounds harsh and unwelcoming."

"If you want, I'd be happy to send it to you so you can read it," he said. "In fact, how about I just read it to you, now?"

"No, just drop it in an email and send it to me; that way I can read it and try to have a visitor's perspective."

"Anything else?"

"The last thing—and maybe I should preface my words by saying that, first, I trust the intentions of the person who visited me. I didn't get the sense that there was any ill will involved. Second, it's never an easy situation to sort out. Still, when I discover pastors abusing the office entrusted to them, I step in and do what I can to get things back on track. You need to know that. And you should also keep in mind the rule of thumb that wherever there are concerns like these, there are probably five more people in your church with the same concerns."

This was a threat. The young pastor took a moment to digest it before re-engaging.

"Again, Bishop," he said. "I don't mean to question you, but I think you may be misinterpreting this person's intentions. You just said that this person told you I changed the whole worship bulletin and made it harder for the people to follow. The impression was that I just kind of went and shuffled everything around in the congregation's worship life without considering or consulting anyone. That's a lie. That's not true."

"Again, John, I don't think this person has any ill will toward you. I think there's a genuine desire to see you succeed. In fact, that's exactly what was said in the conversation, and I encouraged fellowship and follow-through to bring these concerns to a close."

"But, Bishop—"

"—Which gets me back to the third concern," the Bishop interrupted. "The previous pastor was very approachable. I know this because I've known him for a very long time. I hope you realize that to build relationships with the people, you must make yourself available as much as possible, especially in the first year."

"I don't understand," he said. "What have I done to give the impression that I'm not approachable?"

"Well, first of all," he began to explain, "I have a note here which says that it takes you an unusual amount of time to return messages when people call and that you can sometimes be very hard to find during the day when people stop by."

"But that doesn't mean I'm unapproachable," he defended. "That just means I'm busy. And I am. There's a lot going on around the place."

"What are you doing with your time, John?"

"I'm doing what I should be doing."

"Which is?"

"I'm visiting my members and shut-ins. I'm writing sermons, preparing Bible studies, attending meetings, and a whole laundry list of things. I also have a wife and three kids—two more than my predecessor."

"Do the people know everything you do during a typical day?"

"I suppose. I don't know. With all due respect, Bishop," he said attempting dutiful submission. "I tell my secretary where I'm going whenever I leave the building. She knows all my appointments. And if I forget to tell her where I'll be, she has my mobile number. She can always find me. If anyone needs me, they can always find me."

"Well, I hope that's true, John," the Bishop said and sighed. I really do, because this person was concerned enough about this whole situation to drive all the way out here to the district office to meet with me."

"Bishop," the young pastor attempted somewhat sheepishly to encourage. "Could it be that perhaps this person just doesn't like me and would rather have my predecessor serving here instead? Trust me. I get it."

"Oh, no," he said. "I didn't sense that at all. I know for a fact that this person voted in favor of calling you to the church."

"You were told this?"

"Absolutely. And you should know that this person is praying for you and your family regularly."

They're probably praying the imprecatory Psalms, John thought while considering what he could say to help bring the conversation to a close.

"Well," he tried, "I appreciate the heads-up on this, Bishop. I do. And of course, I'll do all I can to serve the people entrusted to my care with love, and to do so prayerfully and faithfully."

"I know you will, John," the Bishop said. "And I appreciate you taking time with me today to chat about these things."

"Should I anticipate receiving a call from this person to reconcile the issues?" he asked.

"Give it some time and see," he answered. "By the way, how're Karen and the kids?"

"It's 'Kim'," he said, "and they're fine."

"I tell you, on the day of judgment people will give account for every careless word they speak..."

Matthew 12:36

SEVEN

A Careless Word

❖

"SO, WHAT DO you think?" he asked with a smile and handed her the key.

"I just love it!" she said, moving around to the driver's side and climbing in.

"I was able to get a pretty good price for our trade-in," he continued and opened the passenger door to join her. "The salesman said that the high mileage might affect its value, but in the end, he made the numbers work for us. The monthly payment is exactly the same as before."

"How about the insurance?"

"That's going up $15 a month," he said, "but I thought that was reasonable."

"That's great," she said, adjusting the van's mirror. "There's so much room for the kids."

"And it only has 55,000 miles," he added. "With the kind of mileage I put on vehicles, it's perfect for us."

She was beaming.

"Did you have Brad look at it?" she asked. "He knows cars better than anyone else."

"Yeah, he checked it out last night before the dealership closed."

"And?"

"And… he looked it over from top to bottom. He even had them put it on the lift so he could get a look from underneath. He said it's a great car."

"You mean no more 'check engine' lights?"

"That's right. No more 'check engine' lights. No more roadside breakdowns. No more duct tape."

"What year is it?" she asked.

"It's only three years old. Not new, but not old."

She started the engine and adjusted the radio.

"I love it," she said. "I can't wait to show the kids."

"Yeah," he said. "They'll be happy that they each get their own seat. No more cramming in like sardines."

"Want to go with me to pick them up from school?"

"I can't," he said. "I need to get back over to the hospital to see Gale. She should be coming out of surgery right about now and I told her this morning that I'd be waiting for her when she made it into a room."

"Okay," she said and closed the driver's door. "I'll see you tonight, then."

He got out and gave the door a gentle push to close it. He turned and tapped on the window. "Call me and tell me what the kids say, okay?" She gave him a thumbs-up and drove away.

He reached into his back pocket to grab his cell phone and dialed the number to the hospital. He figured he'd better call ahead to ensure Gale was out of surgery.

"Not yet," her husband, Don, said. "They're still working on the old bird."

"Okay, then I'm heading to the church to work on some things. Maybe just give me a call when she's out. I should have enough time to get there before she wakes up."

"Will do, Reverend. Thanks for calling."

Over the course of about a half hour, he made a few phone calls, tapped out the concluding paragraphs for the rough draft of Sunday's sermon, and then wrestled unsuccessfully with the network printer to produce a copy.

His phone rang.

"Hello?"

"We need to get a different car," the voice on the other end of the line said flatly.

"What's wrong with the new one?" he asked her.

"Nothing," she said. "It's perfect. Absolutely perfect."

"So, what's the problem?"

"We just need a different car."

"Why?"

"Maybe we can get the dealership to return our old car."

"What are you talking about!" he said beginning to lose his patience. "That car was a piece of junk! It was all but ready to be put in the grave."

"I know," she said. "But maybe we can get it back and then try to keep it running for another year or two."

"It's over twelve years old… and we'll be paying on the credit cards we used to keep it running for the next twelve." Dropping into his office chair, he asked, "What's wrong with the new one?"

"We shouldn't be driving something so nice. It doesn't look right."

"What do you mean it doesn't look right?"

"It just doesn't look right," she said.

"Grace, I'm not taking the car back to the dealership. This is a good thing for our growing family. It's going to help us."

A moment passed. He could tell she was driving with the window down.

"Ginny Schmidt was at the school picking up Jason and Kimberly," she said.

"So?"

"She commented on the new van."

"What did she say?"

Another moment passed. He could hear the wind rasping and popping in the phone's receiver.

"Well, first she asked what happened to the old car. I think she thought it was in the shop or something and that this one was just a rental."

"And?"

"And I told her that you just picked this one up today, that we traded in the other one for this one."

"So, what's the problem?"

"The problem is that she said—she actually said—that she wondered how a guy who only worked one day a week could afford such a nice car."

"You're kidding?"

"She was absolutely serious," she said, replacing her surprise with anger. "I thought she was joking at first," she continued, "but then she said something

89

along the lines that the church must have its priorities mixed up—or as she put it, 'The church must've taken a pretty penny from the mission can for the pastor's new ride.'"

"Wow," was his only word.

"Do you think anyone else will feel the same way?" she asked, her anger becoming a nervous concern again.

"I don't know," he said. "I can't see most folks begrudging the pastor and his family having a reliable car."

"Me either," she said. "And it's not like it's a brand new Porsche. It's a used minivan. But still, I never would have expected that from Ginny."

"Yeah, me either."

"If she's thinking it, then I wonder what others will say. And I know for a fact that she talks to everyone—*everyone*."

"So, what do you want to do?" he asked.

"I don't know. What do you want to do?"

"Well," he said, feeding paper into the printer on his desk, "I can call the dealership and see if we could downgrade a little."

"To what?"

"Maybe there's a sedan on the lot that would work."

"But we need more space…"

"Well, then let's just keep the van," he said, clicking the "print" icon on his screen. The printer gears turned and the feeder grabbed a page. "But I don't want this to be an issue for us," he said. "If you're uncomfortable, we can get something else."

She was quiet. Again, he could hear the road noise.

"Just call the dealership and see what else they have on the lot."

"None is righteous, no, not one..."

Romans 3:10

EIGHT

The Pastor's Kid

❖

HE SOMETIMES WENT to the church with his dad in the evenings. It was, quite often, the only way they could be together.

"You sure you don't just want to go home, Mike?" his Dad asked. "It's a counseling appointment and will be at least an hour. I could call Mom to come and get you."

"That's okay," he said. "I can wait around out here till you're done."

"Are you going to shoot around in the gym?"

"I don't know. Maybe." He had another idea.

"Well, just give me an hour and then how about we stop to get some ice cream on the way home?"

"Sounds good," he said. "Can I drive?"

"Sure," his Dad said and smiled. "Now, get out of here before my appointment shows up. Go practice your free throws."

He wandered down the hallway to one of the meeting rooms and waited.

He knew that the trustees didn't necessarily like him going up there. Still, since the building was like a second home, he'd learned the best way to get onto the roof over the years without being seen. And besides, the last time someone needed to get up there to reset the air conditioning unit, Michael was the one who went.

"Hi, Pastor," he heard two voices say in the hallway.

"Hey, folks," his Dad chimed. "Come on in and have a seat." He waited until his Dad went into his office and closed the door before crossing the hall to the secretary's office. He opened the desk's middle drawer, grabbed the spare master keys, shuffled further down the hallway, and crossed the gymnasium to the basement door.

Flipping through to the maintenance key, he unlocked the door. He bounded down the twenty-one steps in only seven leaps, eventually landing at the bottom with what would have appeared to any unsuspecting bystander as a well-choreographed ricochet and spin-off of the boiler room door at the bottom. This made him laugh every time.

Using the same key as before, he unlocked the deadbolt, pushed the door open, and reached around the doorframe to feel for the light switch, even though light probably wasn't necessary for navigating. He'd done this so many times he could make his way through the room blindfolded— weaving between the furnace and the boxes filled to the brim with old hymnals and ancient Sunday school materials no one wanted to throw out, beneath the low-hanging water pipes, and around the corner to a ladder bolted to the wall and lifting straight up three stories to the padlocked utility door that opened to the roof. He scurried through the maze, took hold of the ladder, and climbed. Once at the top, he plinked the keys one by one until he came to a much smaller key, put it into the lock, turned it, and set free the door. He climbed onto the roof like a submarine captain championing a perfect surfacing.

The sun was just beginning to set over the cornfields behind the church. He could see the flashing red light hanging over the four-way stop in the middle of town. He could see the high school and hear the marching band practicing on the football field. He could see the McDonald's where his best friend Jacob was, at that very moment, taking orders and handing people trays of food. He could see his house, his yard, his mom's car. He could see everything—his town and the entire world beyond it fading into an upland of approaching darkness.

He went to the edge of the building where the roof began its slant and sat down. He put on his headphones, scrolled to his favorite band, and laid back on the roof tiles. They were still warm from the day's sun. He closed his eyes.

It wasn't long before he heard what he thought was a voice calling his name. He sat up and looked around, but didn't see anyone else around. Taking the earbud out of his left ear, he could hear his name being shouted.

"Michael!"

Uh-oh, he thought.

"Michael!" he heard again. "I see you up there! Get off the roof!"

Even though he couldn't tell where the voice was coming from, he knew who it was. It was Mr. Walters, the head trustee, who did not like anyone climbing onto the church's roof.

Michael hunched and ran back to the roof door, climbed in and locked it, and slid down the ladder like a veteran fireman. Dodging the basement obstacles, he hopped through to the boiler room door, locked the deadbolt, and sprinted up the stairs, his ascent matching the same number of leaps as his descent. Mr. Walters was already waiting just beyond the top step.

"I would think," he said before Michael could get a word out, "that of all kids, you would know better."

"Sorry, Mr. Walters."

"Gimme those," he said, taking the keys from Michael's hand. "Just because you're the pastor's kid doesn't mean you can do whatever you want."

"No, I—"

"—Like I said," he started again, except now he was pointing and wagging his finger, "I expect this behavior from the other kids, but not from you. Really, you should know better."

Michael didn't say anything. He just stood and waited for the familiar speech to finish—a prattling reminder as to just how different he was from all of the other kids, how he must be held to a different standard of expectation, and how it reflects poorly upon his family and the church—all of this because his Dad was the pastor.

"Where's your dad, now?"

"He's in a meeting in his office," he said. "I was just hanging around while I waited for him."

"Let's go tell him where I found you," he said, taking Michael's arm.

The boy shrugged away. "He's in a counseling appointment with someone," he said. "We should wait till he's done."

"Oh, no," Mr. Walters affirmed, retaking his arm. "We're going to interrupt his meeting. You're not getting off the hook this time."

"Go tell him yourself," Michael said more intently, jerking his arm away.

"How dare you?!" Mr. Walter's glared.

Michael turned and started down the hallway toward the front doors. Just past the coat racks, he kicked the wall as hard as he could leaving a gaping hole in the drywall near the baseboard. The impact caused the guest registry to fall from its shelf to the floor.

He went outside and sat on the hood of his Dad's car. The sun was much lower than before. And while his view was not as grand as it had been while he was on the roof, his town was before him again—and the entire world beyond it fading into an upland of approaching darkness.

"If anyone thinks he is religious and does not bridle his tongue but deceives his heart, this person's religion is worthless."

James 1:26

NINE

Genie in a Bottle

❖

"IT'S HER, AGAIN," Amy whispered with a stale glare while covering the receiver. "What do you want me to do?"

"Ask her if I can call her back in the morning when I get to the office," he said just as quietly. He'd seen her five times in three days, each appearance being an unannounced visit that consumed a portion of his day that he simply could not afford. In between each of the visits, he'd received four voicemail messages and participated in an equal number of phone conversations that, as with the in-person interactions, taxed his time unnecessarily.

He loved his parish. He loved the people. But with her, he was starting to feel like a genie in a bottle—someone she believed she could summon at will. And her monopoly of his time was only getting worse. Essential tasks were being left undone, he was arriving late to scheduled appointments, and he was grappling with the guilt of stealing time from his family to do the administrative chores required.

"Nancy," Amy said, "he's busy right now and wondering if he might just give you a call in the morning." He could hear the tinny drone of her voice on the phone from across the room.

"Hold on a second," Amy said, turning back to him. "She says it can't wait until morning. She says it's urgent." Giving an exceptionally long but measured exhale, he crossed the kitchen and took the phone from his wife's hand.

"Hi, Nancy," he said. "What's going on?"

"Oh, thank you for taking a minute with me, Pastor," she said. "I know it's late, but I just needed to call and tell you that I did what you said, and I spoke to my father, but he hung up on me before I could finish. What do I do now?"

"Nancy, it's 10:30, and I just got home," he attempted ever-so-gently to explain. "Do you mind if we talk about this tomorrow?"

She continued as though he hadn't said a word.

"I thought that if I explained to him how I was feeling," she said, "he'd understand, and maybe things would get better."

"Nancy—"

"But he hung up on me. How can a father hang up on his own daughter?"

"Nancy—"

"Now, what do I do?"

Knowing full well that he was risking a much longer conversation if he responded with anything other than an insistence that the conversation be continued in the morning, he offered a passing suggestion, "Maybe just give him until morning and then try him again," he urged. "Give him a chance to sleep on what you could say before he hung up."

"You think?"

"Yes, give it until morning. And in the meantime, pray that the Lord will open his heart to listen. That's about all you can do. You can't force him to hear you."

Even though you're sort of forcing me to do both right now, he thought to himself.

"You're right, Pastor," she said, sounding calmer. "I'll try him again tomorrow."

"Sounds like a plan," he said.

"Good night," she returned. "And sorry again for the bother."

"That's okay. Good night, Nancy," and he hung up the phone. But he didn't move from the place where the phone was sitting.

"What are you doing?" Amy asked him. "Isn't it time for bed?"

"I'm just waiting."

"For what?"

"For her to call again."

"But you pushed everything to tomorrow?"

"Doesn't matter," he said, tapping on the table where the phone was resting. "I've talked to her enough to know that this phone is going to ring one more—"

The phone rang.

"—time."

"Don't you dare answer that," Amy said, pointing at him. "You're enabling her. Just turn the ringer off." He was far too tired to disagree with her, so that's exactly what he did.

At the church the following day, he was doing a quick scan of the weekend's service bulletin before leaving for a hospital visitation when he heard the heavy steps of someone on approach in the hallway.

It was Nancy.

"I can't believe you could be so cruel to someone in your church," she said even as she was still coming around the corner and washing into his office. She was breathing rapidly from both her stride and her emotion. "I called you right back last night," she said, "and I know you were there because I'd just talked to you five seconds before."

"Nancy—" he started to say.

"That was really cruel of you to ignore my call," she said, her breath still at a swift pace.

"Nancy, I'm sorry," he said, lifting his hands to calm her. "I went to bed. It was a very long day, and I was so incredibly tired. And you were going to wait—"

"—It was just one last thing, Pastor," she said. "You didn't have a minute more you could chisel from your schedule?"

"Again, Nancy, I'm sorry," he said, attempting to redirect the conversation. "Did you call your dad back yet?"

"No, I didn't call him back yet," she said feverishly. "I'm here trying to understand how you could be so blatantly mean to me."

"Nancy, I wasn't trying to be mean, I was—"

"—Well, be whatever you want, Pastor," she said, turning to leave. "I guess if you don't have time to help the people in your church, then…whatever. Do what you think is right."

"Nancy," he said and followed her out the door. "I just figured we'd finish the conversation today. I didn't mean to offend you."

"I've seen your true colors, Pastor," she said. "I'm sure it won't be long before others do, too."

"Nancy, this really isn't fair," he said, following her to the front door. "Let's go back to my office and sit and talk this through."

"I can't," she said. "I'm already late for work because of this."

"Well," he continued, "maybe give me a call when you have a free moment, and we'll try to sort this out."

"Yeah, maybe," she said, making what she felt was her point. "If I can find the time."

TEN

"Whoever goes about slandering reveals secrets, but he who is trustworthy in spirit keeps a thing covered."

Proverbs 11:13

In Confidence

❖

HE HUNG UP the phone. He actually felt
better. It was good to talk about it, to get the
details out into the open with a friend,
someone he could trust.

Still sitting at the little desk in the corner of the
family room below the crucifix, he offered a quick
prayer of thanksgiving to the Lord. He thanked Him
for his family, for the opportunity to be His servant
among the people, for the guidance and protection
He had provided for so long, for the listening ear of
a singular friend and the voice of that same brother

reminding him that he wasn't alone in the fray—
giving to him the Good News of salvation through
the death of Christ and reminding him that no matter
how the Devil might try to convince him otherwise,
God was not at war with him. Through faith in Jesus,
the war between God and man was over.

He went to bed that night and slept much more
soundly than any of the previous nights of the past
six months.

The next day was filled with all the same
challenges. Yet, as he moved from task to task,
meeting to meeting, visitation to visitation, he felt
more resilient—more refreshed.

He was finally feeling as though things could get
better.

Having just finished leading a worship service at
the local assisted living home, he was gently laying
his vestments into the backseat of his car when his
mobile phone pinged. It was a text message from a
friend, a former seminary classmate, someone he'd
not spoken with in quite some time. And although the
two may not have had the opportunity over the past
year to visit, he was glad to see his name appear on
the screen.

"You doing okay?" the message read.

He was surprised by the question. The two hadn't
spoken since they'd seen one another last year at the

112

seminary's annual theological conference. It was an unexpected greeting.

"Yeah, I'm fine," he typed in response. "How about you? Things are well?"

"I'm fine," pinged another note. "I was just worried about you. Hoping you're okay."

"Busy as usual. Lots going on around here," he returned and then closed the door to the back seat. Waiting for the next response, he opened the driver-side door and sat down, his feet still out of the car and resting on the pavement.

"Are you going to be able to make it down to the conference this year?" came another note. "Would be great to see you."

"Probably not. But I'm hoping for next year, God willing."

"You should try for this year if you can. You're not that far away, and a year is a long time, my friend."

He started to type, but another message arrived before he could finish.

"All the guys are here. We're at The Red Raven having an afternoon beer."

"Sounds like fun. Have one for me."

"The rest of the afternoon sessions didn't look all that interesting, so a few of us figured we'd skip out and reminisce. LOL."

"Who's there with you?"

"Steve, Kurt, John, and Will. Their wives are here, too, but they wanted a different table for themselves. They're right next to us complaining that a table full of clergymen shouldn't be talking so loudly."

"Tell everyone I said hello."

"Will do. Steve just told us he talked to you last night, and things weren't going well for you right now. Anything I can do to help?"

His stomach plunged.

"What did he tell you?"

"Just that you've been struggling with the people there. Sounds like the place is full of haters who don't appreciate their pastor."

"That's not true. There are many good folks here showing us a lot of love. But there's a handful making the work challenging." He was speaking truthfully. He knew that most of his flock loved and appreciated him and were working alongside him to exercise church discipline among those attempting to drive him out through clandestine efforts.

He sat for a moment and then started to type, but it became apparent that his friend could send texts much more swiftly than he did.

"Steve said that you're thinking about quitting the ministry."

"He did?"

"Don't even think about doing that, brother. We'll all drive up there and smack you."

"What else did he say?"

"He said Janie already transferred herself and the kids to another church in the area. Did she really? It sounds like she's had enough of those people. Are you two okay?"

"I can't believe…" he started to type but erased it. Another message landed before him.

"At least you guys are seeing a counselor. That's smart. Stick together."

He started to type again but was interrupted.

"The girls at the other table said to tell Janie hello and that they're praying for her."

"Janie and I are fine. Don't worry. We're in this together."

"That's good. She needs to have your back. I don't think Mary would have transferred out if I were in the same situation. How did the people respond when she did it?"

"You don't know all the details," he managed to type and send. "It's complicated."

"I got you. Mary just said that if Janie needs someone to talk to that, she just needs to call."

"Where's Steve right now?"

"He's up at the bar waiting for the beer."

"Do me a favor, will you?"

"Sure. Anything, buddy."

"When Steve gets back to the table—and make sure the wives are listening—remind him that I asked him to keep everything I shared in confidence, and then let him know that I won't be making that mistake again."

The messages stopped.

Several minutes passed before he finally turned and tossed his phone into the passenger seat. Lifting himself the rest of the way into the car and closing the door, he heard another ping just as he put his key into the ignition.

"Hey, brother," the new thread began. "It's Steve. Do you mind if I give you a quick call?"

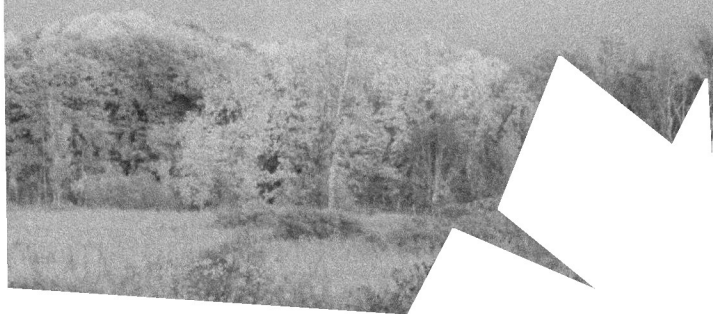

A Last Word

A LAST WORD

❖

THE LAST WORD needn't be lengthy.
There are two things in particular that serve to maintain the climate described in the stories you've just read.

The first is the immobilizing bondage to *fear*.

For a pastor who has become the target of abuse, it isn't uncommon to experience feelings of extreme inadequacy toward God, the congregation, and his family. There is the feeling that he has fallen far short of his vow to the Lord, has failed to meet the needs of the people in his care, and has been wholly insufficient in providing for the health and safety of his family.

Staring into the frightful eyes of self-doubt, fear is born.

As a result of such anxiety, the pastor may find himself inclined to deal with the situation alone—maintaining silence because he fears that any attempt to bring to light the furtive words and actions leveled against him (most often by well-respected members) will almost certainly fall upon deaf ears, or, quite simply, be received as implausibly outlandish and a symptom of a personal deficiency such as paranoia or another personality disorder.

For a parishioner, stepping forward to both speak and act in defense of an abused pastor means being willing to assume into oneself the same assaults to body, soul, spirit, and reputation that he is experiencing. It means coupling such pain with the equally distressing forecast of forfeiting longtime personal relationships.

Faced with such terrifying prospects, fear is certainly to be expected.

The second is the crippling fetter of *ignorance*.

God is at work for the good of those who love Him. One way He so generously dispenses His love is through helpers (Hebrews 10:25; Philippians 2:4; Romans 12:13; Matthew 25:35-39). Pastors must become aware of the support services available to them, not only through their congregation and denominational structures but also among the community of the Christian Church at large. Take for example the following organizations:

ShepherdsCanyonRetreat.org
GracePlaceWellness.org
Doxology.us
BroomTreeMinistries.org
PastorCare.org

The above regenerative stanchions are all examples of reputable organizations in place to provide a variety of help for ministers suffering from abuse, exhaustion, doubt, and so many other struggles unique to pastoral ministry.

Relative to parishioners, ignorance of the pastor's personal needs may be overcome by establishing a support mechanism within the congregation's framework designed to keep a finger on the pulse of his mental, physical, and spiritual well-being. A somewhat simplified example of this might be for an appropriate church board to be charged with adding to its monthly agenda a regular item entitled "Health and Well-being." During this time, as deemed appropriate (and within the comfortable boundaries of confidentiality), the pastor should be encouraged to speak freely about anything causing him or his family any undue difficulty or grief. Providing he takes advantage of the platform, such dialogue can be a therapeutic means for early detection of issues that have the potential to become devastating hindrances to his personal life and public ministry. It should also be noted that the time together in discussion may also be an opportunity for him to share those occasional moments of joy that not only bring delight to his labor but serve to highlight God's loving-kindness at work among the congregation and community.

And so, without losing sight of where it was that we began, to conclude by acknowledging that fear and ignorance are formidable foes to both pastor and parishioner is for us to admit that to overcome such adversaries, unearthly courage is required—the kind that only Christ can give.

Remember, He has already provided it by way of His Gospel.

And no matter the mortal endpoint to the story, one of the inherent promises of God located in the all-sufficient sacrifice of His Son on the cross is that

He will preserve you according to His holy will, and you will persevere (John 14:27; 16:33).

God grant you such faith, by the power of His Holy Spirit, to believe this.

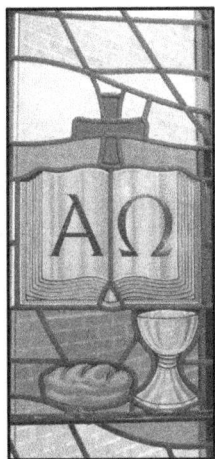

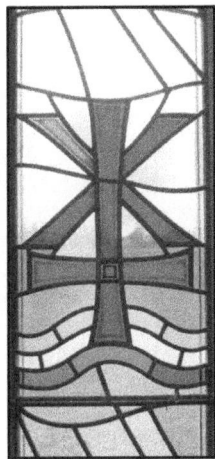